HEALTH & FITNESS

AMAZING SUGGESTIONS YOU SHOULD KNOW

By Charles Naylor

Chapter 1 ; Health

Health is not just the absence of disease or disability; it is a state of total physical, mental, and social well-being. Maintaining one's physical condition and taking precautions to lower the risk of contracting various diseases constitutes being healthy. Health is the body's innate capacity to adjust to both physical and psychological changes that it encounters. Living a healthy lifestyle should be a part of your whole philosophy because it can help prevent chronic illnesses and long-term diseases. It's crucial for your self-esteem and self-image to feel good about yourself and to take care of your physical well-being. Physical, emotional, social, intellectual, and spiritual health are the five fundamental facets of individual well-being. None of these areas must be ignored if one is to be regarded as "well.". The single most crucial thing you can do for your health is to exercise frequently, ideally every day. Exercise reduces the risk of heart disease, stroke, diabetes, dementia, depression, and many malignancies over the long term while also enhancing mood, improving sleep, and controlling hunger in the near term.

Physical Health:

Physical health can be described as the body functioning normally on all levels, biological processes running normally to ensure individual survival and reproduction, a dynamic balance between the body's functions and the environment, engagement in social activities and work that benefits society, the performance of basic social tasks, the absence of diseases, uncomfortable conditions, and changes, and the body's capacity to adapt to the constantly shifting environmental conditions.

Physical exercise

Regular exercise is necessary for physical health. A physically fit individual creates exercise regimens that they can stick to. These ought to be engaging pursuits that may be incorporated into everyday life. Among them is taking part in an organized sport like tennis or golf. It might also incorporate more relaxed pursuits like strolls, bike rides, or visits to the gym. Regular repetition of the activity is more likely if it is fun and convenient. Repetition regularly improves physical wellness.

Regular exercise has an effect not only on the body but also on the brain. Regular exercise can help to reduce anxiety. It can hone your ability to reason and make decisions. Even better sleep for people may result from it.

Regular physical activity can also lower your risk of getting sick. Exercise for 150 minutes a week reduces the risk of cardiovascular diseases like heart disease and stroke. Additionally, it can reduce the risk of diseases like type 2 diabetes and even some types of cancer. Regular physical activity can help to maintain a chronic condition, even if the person already has it. A person can maintain a healthy weight, have stronger bones, and have stronger muscles by engaging in regular physical activity. The health of all of these things can be enhanced.

Factors Affecting Physical Health
The primary areas of physical health can be addressed by lifestyle choices in the ways listed below:

Physical activity is something that most healthy kids and adults should do every day. This should include both unstructured exercise and relaxing physical activities. Walking, riding, and hiking are a few examples of leisurely physical activity. Strength training, running, and sports are a few examples of more structured kinds of exercise.

Diet and nutrition: A well-balanced diet should include a variety of vitamins, minerals, proteins, and carbohydrates. Only a trained health practitioner should be in charge of restricting any particular nutrition. Regular fluid intake is recommended, ideally in the form of pure water. Daily meals and snacks should be eaten, and portion quantities should be reasonable.

Drugs and alcohol: Consuming these substances in moderation or avoiding them altogether is advised. Consider total abstinence from these substances if you have addictive tendencies or other health concerns.

Medical self-care: The essentials, such as bandages, lozenges, and over-the-counter painkillers, should be available at home. Primary care should be used for persistent coughing, fevers, or other illnesses. When signs and symptoms are serious or life-threatening, emergency care should be sought.

While regular exercise is vital for physical health, getting enough rest is equally critical. The body can be refreshed by taking brief naps or relaxing for some time. Sleep should last between seven and nine hours in a peaceful, dark setting. A healthcare provider may need to be consulted when the amount or quality of sleep is consistently substantially shorter or longer than this.

Physical Health Evaluations

You may already be aware of the many methods for evaluating physical health if you've recently seen a doctor or personal trainer. Aspects of physical health can be tested using the following measurements:

General evaluations: reflex tests, weight, and body mass index (BMI).
Tests for blood pressure, cholesterol, and blood sugar are included in assessments of disease risk factors.

Body composition (% of body fat), flexibility, muscular strength, and endurance tests are all included in fitness examinations.

How do you maintain your physical well-being?

Several crucial elements can be incorporated into life to control physical wellness. These include regular physical activity, healthy eating, rest, decent cleanliness, and frequent preventative care.

What types of physical health are examples of?

Both the absence of illness and general body soundness are components of physical health. A regular schedule that includes a variety of activities might promote wellness. Stretching exercises, muscle- and bone-building exercises, and cardiovascular exercises are a few of these.

Emotional/mental Health;

Emotional health is a state of positive psychological functioning. It is possible to conceptualize it as a continuation of mental health; it is the "optimal functioning" conclusion of the ideas, emotions, and actions that constitute both our inner and outward worlds. Through both the highs and lows of life, it involves an overall experience of wellness in what we think, feel, and do.

When people talk about mental health, they may also be referring to ideas like emotional health and well-being. The phrases "emotional health" and "mental health" are interchangeable. However, there is frequently a distinction between the two. The term "mental health" refers to a state of being that ranges from full function to crippling mental illness and is related to the brain/mind, thoughts, feelings, and behaviors. In contrast, emotional health relates to well-being and the way one perceives and leads a healthy life.

Behaviors that pertain to the mind or brain are included in mental health. Associated issues commonly arise as a result of a chemical imbalance in the brain. These problems could involve:

Anxiety

Depression

Bipolar illness

erratic eating

PTSD

Several factors can cause a chemical imbalance in the brain. A natural chemical imbalance that results in a mental health condition is one way. Usually, this issue might develop if the mental illness runs in the family. A chemical imbalance can also develop when a person uses medicines that change their perception.

On the other hand, emotional health addresses personal issues. People who experience stressful or unfortunate life situations are more likely to acquire problems in the future.

The Relationship Between Emotional and Mental Health

Even though emotional and mental health is two distinct concepts, they are nevertheless linked. Without mental health care, people's emotions may go out of control. Purely concentrating on emotional well-being throws the mind off balance, making it challenging to carry out daily tasks. Treatments for emotional and mental health play a part in supporting patients during rehabilitation.

How to Spot Someone Who Is Having Mental or Emotional Issues

People who battle with emotional or mental health concerns may experience a variety of symptoms. Even though it is conceivable for someone to experience both simultaneously, one is usually the root cause. How can they differentiate between the two, though?

Mentally ill individuals may behave in ways that cause them to distance themselves from friends and family. This makes it more difficult to comprehend their issues. Healthy boundaries can be difficult for those with emotional problems, and they may also have codependency issues with their loved ones.

Encourage a loved one to seek help if you believe they are experiencing mental or emotional distress. It can enhance their general health and way of life.

For overall well-being, managing one's mental and emotional health is important.

During treatment, it's crucial to successfully manage both emotional and mental processes. This improves general health and addresses a variety of issues, *including*:

Depression

Anger

Fear

Anxiety

Stress

Worry

Social Health:

Our capacity to engage in meaningful interpersonal interactions is referred to as our social health. It also has to do with how well we can adjust to social settings. Our ability to build satisfying interpersonal interactions with others as well as our mental and physical health are all affected by our social ties. It also has to do with your capacity for easy social adjustment and proper behavior across a range of contexts. Relationships between spouses, coworkers, and acquaintances can all be fruitful. Each of these connections should be characterized by effective communication, empathy for others, and a feeling of responsibility... On the other hand, personality traits like withdrawal, resentment, or selfishness might be detrimental to your social health. Overall, one of the biggest dangers to a strong relationship is stress. Stress should be addressed using tried-and-true methods like frequent exercise, deep breathing, and encouraging self-talk.

Sociologists have shown a connection between social connections and health outcomes throughout time. Studies have shown that the quantity and quality of social contacts have both immediate and long-term implications on our health.

Intellectual

The pursuit of mental wellness, ongoing intellectual development, and lifelong creativity is referred to as intellectual health or intellectual wellness. Continued education, problem-solving practice, linguistic skill development, keeping up with social and political concerns, and reading books, periodicals, and newspapers are some examples of this.

Spiritual Health;

What cannot be classified as a component of the body or the mind is the spirit. The three are interconnected and have an impact on one another. You can aid in the healing process by developing your spiritual life. While spirituality may not be able to heal you, it can help you manage the suffering and challenges that come with sickness. When you are at peace with life, you are in good spiritual health. It occurs when you can find consolation and hope during the most trying of circumstances. You can get assistance from it as you fully enjoy life. For each person, spirituality is distinct.

It may be simple to lose your spiritual health when dealing with a chronic illness. You might occasionally feel tempted to abandon your convictions. It's crucial to bear in mind that managing your physical health is made easier by maintaining a good spiritual life. You can deal with any problems that may occur with your physical health by focusing on your spiritual life. Our beings are whole. Balance can help us stay healthy and recuperate.

You might wish to ask yourself the following questions if your spiritual health is a problem for you:

What fills me with the most satisfaction?
What time of day do I feel the most a part of the world?
Where do I get my inner strength from?
What do I do when I'm feeling complete?
You might find the solutions to your inner peace by using the questions above. You can give your body more strength for healing if you can find inner calm. Peace of mind is necessary for our physical bodies. They can thus have some downtime to relax and heal. This is just another way that the state of our spiritual health might influence how we heal.

Chapter 2; The significance of health

- The benefits of good health include increased longevity.

A person's daily schedule would be impacted by living an unhealthy lifestyle. The body becomes more fit and healthy and can live longer when it receives the right nutrients.

- Prevent diseases

The key to living a healthy life is having a strong immune system that can fend off many illnesses. The immune system serves as the body's natural defensive system against invaders that could harm it. For complete well-being, it is crucial to maintain both physical and mental health.

- Improve mental health

Poor mental health would be the effect of living an unhealthy lifestyle. The mind would be calmed and one's mood would be lifted by adopting a healthy lifestyle.

Only when a person is a content in their minds would they work effectively. Physical and mental wellness are both crucial.

- Lead a productive life

A healthy individual would contribute to their society and country. A person is only regarded as healthy if they are free of any diseases. They might then provide better service as a result.

- Financial benefits

Medical costs are increasing in price. Only by making early investments in one's health can one avoid or lessen the severity of illness development.

They can lower their risk of being hospitalized and cut down on the cost of medical care by maintaining good health.

Chapter 3; Fitness

Fitness is described as "the ability to meet the demands of the environment" or "the ability to perform daily activities with optimal performance, endurance, and strength with the management of disease, fatigue, and stress and reduced sedentary behavior." Cardiovascular functioning is also referred to as fitness, and it is enhanced by aerobic activities that get your heart and lungs pumping more quickly. Balance, flexibility, and muscle strength are also included. Stress can be reduced by participating in sports. A mental benefit is increased self-assurance.

Fitness-related activities;

- Walking.

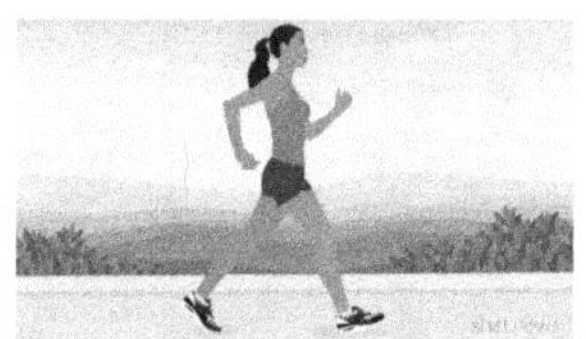

- Dancing.

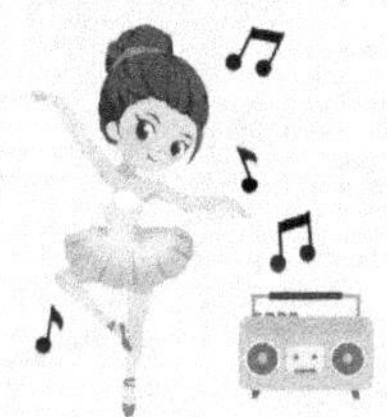

- Swimming.

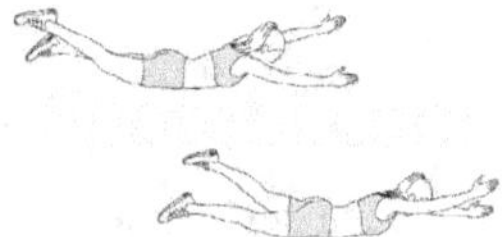

- Water aerobics.

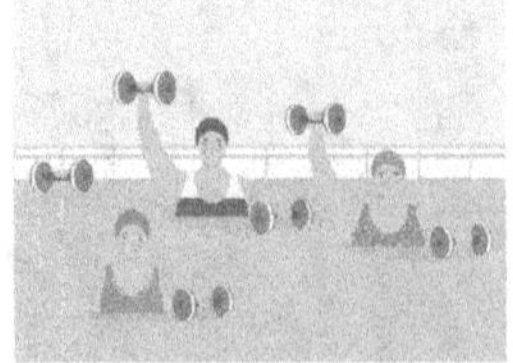

- Jogging and running.

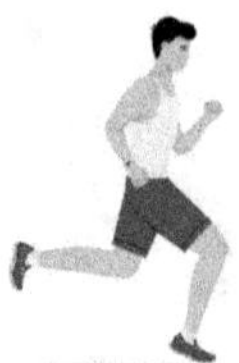

- Aerobic exercise classes.

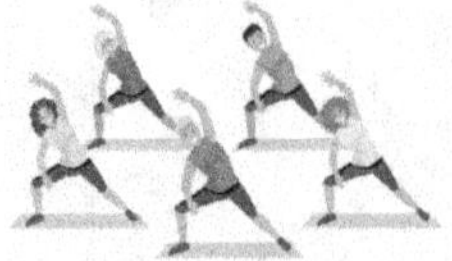

- Bicycle riding (stationary or on a path)

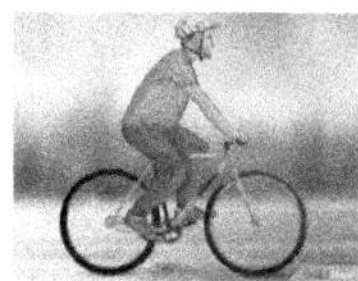

- Some gardening activities, such as raking and pushing a lawn mower.

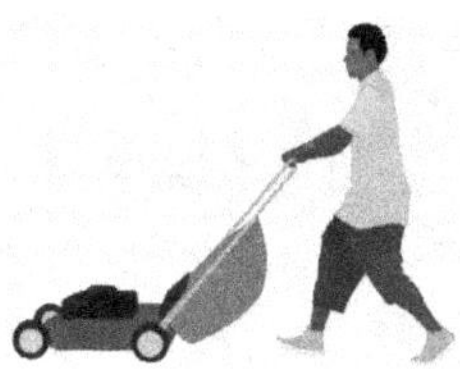

chapter 4; Disparities between fitness and health

The majority of people think that being fit and being healthy is the same thing. They may be distinct states of physical entities. Both being extremely healthy and having a poor level of fitness are possible. The best results come from attempting to strike a balance between the two, which necessitates our understanding of the distinction between fitness and health.

So let's explain the distinction. The World Health Organization defines health as a condition of the whole physical, mental, and social well-being and not just the absence of disease or disability. It encompasses healthy aging, long life, high quality of life, absence of discomfort, etc.

On the other hand, fitness is described as a collection of qualities people possess or attain that have to do with their capacity to engage in physical activity. When considering fitness levels, the following elements must be taken into account because fitness is made up of many different parts:

- The capacity of your body to use and transport oxygen to your body is known as endurance (cardiovascular and cardio-respiratory).
- Your body's capacity to store, process, and use energy is known as stamina (muscular endurance).
- Strength is the capacity of a muscular unit or your body as a whole to exert force.

- Flexibility is the capacity to increase a joint's range of motion

- Power is the capacity of your muscles to exert the greatest amount of force in the shortest amount of time.
- Speed is the capacity to reduce the time it takes you to complete an activity or motion.
- The capacity to blend multiple movement patterns into a single, distinctive movement.
- Accuracy: The capacity to guide movement in a certain direction or degree.
- Agility is the capacity to transition quickly from one movement to another.
- Balance is the capacity to manage your body's center of gravity concerning your support structure.

Fitness includes any type of activity that activates the body's systems and keeps them in a certain state. On the other hand, health involves every bodily system and can only be attained by leading a healthy lifestyle. For instance, no amount of exercise could ever undo the harm caused by a client's lifestyle if they disclose to me that they have neglected to eat appropriately, disregarded the fat content, and consumed primarily processed foods. Exercise won't repair immune system damage or weakness brought on by nutrient-poor meals, nor will it reverse the effects of toxins. Only healthy eating can promote good health. Of course, if it becomes a way of life, exercise may both support and improve health. Our everyday dietary choices, which number thousands, have a significant impact on our health.

Ask yourself this straightforward question as you move forward on your health path, or if you are just getting started again: "Am I on the road to becoming fit and healthy, or just fit?" If "just fit" is your response, consider combining more wellness facets into a larger strategy centered on the integration of physical, mental, emotional, and spiritual health.

Ask yourself what you can do to accomplish more and live life to the fullest if it is just healthy to stop seeing the doctor. Being healthy is nice, but what good is it if you can't take a vacation or go up the stairs without being out of breath? Make sure you are addressing both sides of the issue by speaking with your exercise physiologist and setting goals for both health and fitness/performance. then take a step back and observe your success.

Chapter 5; Ways to enhance your fitness

It's simple to start being active, and you may start at any time. Physical activity is anything that gets you moving, and it is good for you no matter your age. Encourage yourself to work on your fitness.

Motivating yourself could be challenging, especially if it's chilly and rainy outside. However, you may work out and be active anyplace, including at home, at work, or outside.

Choose a reason for becoming more active

Why are you exercising, you could ask? You can wish to feel good, get more rest, have more energy, be stronger, develop muscle tone and flexibility, or just have more energy.

Set goals and achieve it

Make a target that you can actually achieve. To keep track of your progress, keep a journal, a chart, or use an internet application. A pedometer or a health app on your phone can be used to track your steps. Enjoy the task and keep your pace gradual.

Don't beat yourself up

Everybody experiences unpleasant days where they may decide to skip some or all of the activities. Ignore it and resume your course the following day.

Give yourself a treat

Give yourself a reward, preferably a healthy one, when you reach goals or take steps in that direction.

Choose an activity that you enjoy

Pick pastimes you enjoy. Variety is important; if you grow bored with one hobby, switch to another one.

Try to do some activity on most days of the week

The majority of us juggle our busy schedules with our work and family responsibilities. If you allocate a specific time for your daily routine, it will become more active.

Get support

Go walking or jogging with friends, colleagues or family to make it more enjoyable and motivate you. Join a club or online community to track your progress.

Starting your fitness habit

Any action is preferable to none, no matter your age or skill level.

Remember that:

• You can achieve your target of 30 minutes per day by exercising for 10 minutes at a time.

• Select activities that are appropriate for you and seek guidance from your doctor.

• Space out your tasks across the day and the week.

• include exercises that improve physical stamina and strength 2–3 days per week

Aim for moderately intense exercise. Your heart rate will increase with moderate exercise, and you'll also feel warmer and breathe more quickly.

For instance:

• 15 minutes for a mile while walking quickly

• Aquatic exercises

• Cycling at a pace less than ten miles per hour

• dancing

• standard gardening

To increase the health advantages by two times, try working your way up to strenuous levels of activity. Running, playing football, or dancing vigorously for 75 minutes had equivalent health advantages as 150 minutes of moderate exercise.

Activity for your age

- Depending on your age, you should try to achieve a particular level of activity:
- Children and adolescents should engage in at least 60 minutes of moderate-intensity activity each day, and adults should engage in at least 30 minutes of the same. 5-day workweek
- Older adults should engage in moderate-intensity exercise five days a week for at least 30 minutes.
- Start small and work your way up to these levels if you are unable to achieve these targets.

- A balanced diet is one that includes a variety of meals in the right amounts and ratios to meet one's needs for calories, proteins, minerals, vitamins, and other nutrients while also leaving a tiny amount of room for extra nutrients to last through the brief period of leanness. A healthy diet is one that enhances or maintains general health.

- Active way of life – An active way of life involves regular physical activity. An active lifestyle includes any activity that gets you moving.

Exercise includes activities like walking and weightlifting. It also comprises engaging in sports. Exercise vs. yoga during a workout or with yoga. Yoga places more of an emphasis on sustained postures and muscle relaxation. Yoga is described as "a calm and relaxed condition." The breathing is coordinated, and the motions are calm and controlled. The focus of regular exercise is on movement and placing stress on the muscles.

- Limit your intake of fatty foods, such as nuts and vegetable oil. Avocado, peanut butter, olive oil, and so forth.

- Avoid missing meals; doing so might have a detrimental effect on your health if it becomes a habit. Regularly skipping meals can prevent your body from operating or performing to its full potential. Regularly skipping meals can increase stress and leave the body with insufficient energy to function.

- Refrain from using narcotics, alcohol, and tobacco products. Alcohol contains ethanol, a colorless volatile flammable liquid that is a depressant in alcoholic beverages as well as a solvent and fuel. Alone, ethanol consumption can result in death. Excessive alcohol consumption can cause chronic illnesses such heart disease, stroke, liver disease, high blood pressure, breast cancer, throat cancer, and other illnesses that may not be mentioned in this book. Smoking damages almost every organ in the body because it causes you to breathe in and out the gases from burning plant material. Smoking can lead to a variety of illnesses, including heart disease, cancer, diabetes, infections, vision loss, breathing difficulties, and other issues that may not be covered in this book. Drug abuse or overuse can result in death or health problems.

Chapter 6; Bring easy lifestyle suggestions with you

While coffee is fantastic, its ideal to rehydrate with a full glass of water first thing in the morning. Drinking water early thing in the morning can help with digestion, skin health, and vitality.

Climb stairs

The stairs are a simple method to add a little extra physical activity to your daily life instead of using the elevator. While you're doing it, your legs and core are strengthened and toned as well!

Put half your food on vegetables.

Making half your plate of food vegetables at each meal is a quick trick for healthy eating (and portion control). The vegetables are a rich source of phytonutrients, vital vitamins, and other nutrients for good health and long life. They also serve to promote digestion (i.e., keep you regular!) and keep you feeling fuller for a longer period of time because they are high in fiber.

Purchase a fitness monitor and count your steps.

A simple approach to make sure you're getting enough exercise each day is to track your steps with a fitness tracker (like a Fitbit or Apple Watch). Aiming for 10,000 steps each day provides considerable advantages for both physical and mental health. A fitness tracker will also remind you to walk 250 steps every hour, which is another crucial health indicator (see tip #9 for more information). Here are some of our top picks for smartwatch fitness trackers for 2021.

Use less hazardous household cleaning products

Traditional household cleaners contain a lot of dangerous chemicals that are bad for our health and the health of our children and pets. It's easy to decrease your exposure to environmental contaminants in your home by making the switch to healthier substitutes. For a comprehensive list of suggestions and information on how to select safer household cleaning products, see our Healthy Cleaning Guide.

Make use of nontoxic personal care and skincare products.

Conventional skincare and personal care products contain hazardous substances that we shouldn't frequently let to enter our body's main organ, just like traditional cleaning products. Use non-toxic personal care and beauty items to lessen the toxic load on your body (see our specific recommendations on deodorant, sunscreen, and green beauty products).

every day, take a probiotic.

Digestion, skin health, immunity, mental health, and other aspects of health are significantly impacted by maintaining a healthy gut. One of the simplest things you can do to improve your gut health is to take a daily probiotic with a glass of water every morning (which, in turn, boosts overall health in many ways too). Learn more about the advantages of probiotics for your health (and how to incorporate them into your diet) and purchase our top probiotic supplement here.

Consume actual food

Eat as much actual food as you can, preferably from items your grandma would know or those you would find in your own cupboard. Sorry, but this eliminates the majority of packaged foods. This is somewhat different from advising you to consume solely "health foods," many of which are becoming more and more processed. Unprocessed foods like an apple, a cucumber, soybeans, or a steak are examples of "real food," as are foods that have been only minimally processed from one (or a few) real-food constituents, such as butter, olive oil, yogurt, tofu, etc. In other words, choose foods that you could make at home and stay away from those that require special laboratory equipment.

get up and move around for a minute or two every 30 minutes while working to counteract the negative effects of prolonged sitting, such as at a desk job.

Take daily sun exposure

Sunlight is one of our finest sources of vitamin D, which is one of the nutrients that is most crucial for overall health. Attempt to spend at least 30 minutes each day outside, especially in the late afternoon without the use of sunscreen (read more about that here). Where you reside, the winters don't get much sunlight? It might be beneficial to take a vitamin D supplement or eat foods that naturally contain this nutrient.

Put indoor plants all throughout your house.

Research has shown that indoor plants can increase mood, creativity, and problem-solving skills as well as aid to purify the air (which, regrettably, probably needs to be done!).

daily perspiration

Whether it's through hot yoga, dancing, bicycling, running, or any other form of physical activity you enjoy, try to work up a sweat at least once a day. For more workout suggestions, advice on incorporating regular physical activity into your daily life, and a printable fitness planner you can use to create your own personalized fitness plan to remain on track, check out our fitness guide.

Drink a green smoothie every day

Green smoothies make it simple to get your daily recommended amount of greens as a snack or quick meal on the road. For some of our favorite starting green smoothie recipe ideas, browse our collection of healthy (and veggie-packed!) smoothie recipes.

Work hard and show kindness

Enough already!

Develop a positive outlook

"Your attitude is the only thing that separates a good day from a poor day." True, attitude is everything. Develop a positive attitude by identifying your negative thought patterns and replacing them with good ones. Here are some more tools for a good mindset.

Obtain adequate rest

Adults typically require 7-9 hours of sleep per night. But sleep quality is just as important as quantity! Follow our recommendations for achieving good sleep, including keeping your bedroom chilly at night and avoiding blue light after sunset.

Establish a wholesome morning ritual to start the day.

Starting each day with rewarding activities will help you feel motivated, relaxed, productive, or any other way you choose to feel. Check out our list of suggestions for creating a wholesome morning ritual to get your day off to a good start!

consume a rainbow

Try to eat something from each color of the rainbow every day. (Only natural colors; no Skittles. To keep track, fill out and print our free Eat the Rainbow weekly and daily tracker.

Use tooth floss.

For both dental and general wellness, floss your teeth every day. Daily flossing not only keeps your teeth and gums healthy, but it also promotes immunity and heart health.

Take some alone time

Knowing and staying in touch with who you are on a regular basis is beneficial because we are all continually evolving. You can live your most purposeful life by checking in with yourself during your alone time to see how you're doing and what you want. As a healthy way to spend time alone, some people like hiking, going for walks or runs, practicing meditation, or even lying in the sun.

Do things you find enjoyable.

Doing something you enjoy doing every day is something that is frequently forgotten as a crucial component of healthy life. Reserve time each day to spend doing things you particularly enjoy, whether that's exercising, baking, creating, reading a book, or watching TV.

Whenever feasible, seek organic food

We'll allow that more in-depth post linked do the talking and just remind you to choose organic foods whenever possible because there are a ton of health, environmental, and social benefits to do so. They are better for the environment, your health, and the farmworkers who grow your food.

A teaspoon of apple cider vinegar prevents illness

Everything is cured by apple cider vinegar, or almost everything. A teaspoon of apple cider vinegar in a glass of water can help with digestion, bloating relief, immunity-boosting, blood sugar regulation, and other things. We advise using raw, organic apple cider vinegar without filtering.

Laugh a lot.

It's true that smiling improves both your physical and emotional health, so try to smile as frequently as you can throughout the day.

strive to conquer your fears

We are held back by our fears and are unable to live life to the fullest. Recognize your fears and take action to get over them. (One illustration of this is conquering your fear of public speaking to gain access to new opportunities in both your professional and personal life.)

make a desk chair out of a yoga ball.

Use a yoga ball as a desk chair to improve your core and protect your back, shoulders, and neck.

Take care of yourself by managing your stress.

Your physical and emotional health are both negatively impacted by persistent stress. Learn your stress releases (the things that can help you feel calm when you're anxious) and your stress triggers (the things that cause you stress, either rapidly or over time), so you can manage stress and keep healthy levels.

Intermittent fasting may help people lose weight

Since constraints are unpleasant, we don't really enjoy dieting, yet intermittent fasting is more of an eating routine than a diet. It offers a number of noteworthy health advantages, including the ability to speed up metabolism to aid in weight loss, reduce inflammation, and improve longevity.

After each alcoholic beverage, sip a glass of water.
No, we won't advise you to abstain from drinking (but you are more than welcome to do so!). If done responsibly, moderate alcohol consumption can be a component of a "healthy" lifestyle. A glass of water after each alcoholic beverage aids in alcohol detoxification, slows down alcohol consumption, and keeps you hydrated (essential for avoiding hangovers!).

Show gratitude
Every day, try to be grateful. You can do this in the morning, at night, or even during your lunch break at work. Here are some of our favorite gratitude-inspiring ideas, along with a list of the positive effects frequent thankfulness practice has on both your physical and emotional health.

A short stroll around the block is preferable to no stroll at all.
Even a small amount of effort is preferable than doing nothing at all when it comes to leading a healthy lifestyle. Take a quick walk around the block if you want to go for a walk but don't have time for your usual hour-long stroll. Better than not walking at all is a 5-minute stroll!